Terms and Conditions

LEGAL NOTICE

The Publisher has strived to be as accurate and complete as possible in the creation of this report, notwithstanding the fact that he does not warrant or represent at any time that the contents within are accurate due to the rapidly changing nature of the Internet.

While all attempts have been made to verify information provided in this publication, the Publisher assumes no responsibility for errors, omissions, or contrary interpretation of the subject matter herein. Any perceived slights of specific persons, peoples, or organizations are unintentional.

In practical advice books, like anything else in life, there are no guarantees of income made. Readers are cautioned to reply on their own judgment about their individual circumstances to act accordingly.

This book is not intended for use as a source of legal, business, accounting or financial advice. All readers are advised to seek services of competent professionals in legal, business, accounting and finance fields.

You are encouraged to print this book for easy reading.

Table Of Contents

Foreword

Sleep is a constantly recurring event characterized by reduced or absent consciousness. A state of relatively reduced sensory activity, Sleep is believed to be as important as being awake. It is the time where both the body and the mind recuperate from all the stress it has experienced throughout the day. Get all the info you need here.

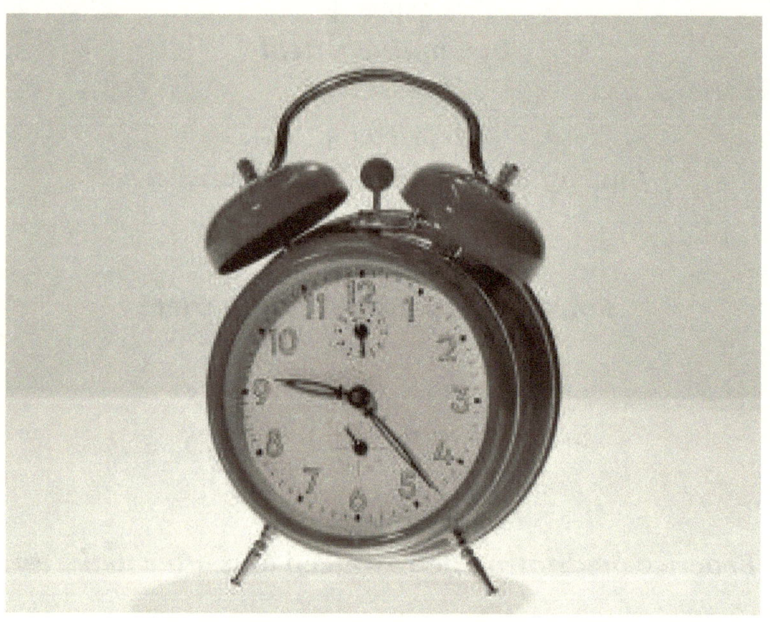

Wake Up Now!
Introduction: Sleep and How it Works

Chapter 1:

Introduction

Synopsis

In sleep, all the voluntary muscles remain inactive and involuntary muscles functions are reduced. In other words, it is like switching off a machine or placing it in idle mode to allow the machines to cool off and prevent damage. It is mostly done at night where hormone levels are at the lowest.

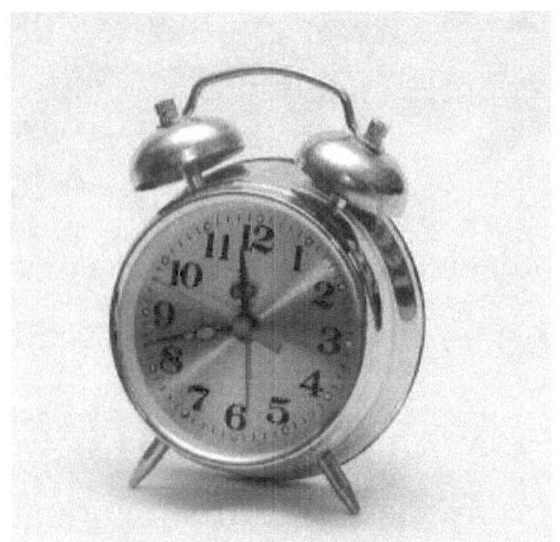

How Sleep Works

A person's sleep can be affected by a lot of factors one of these factors include the circadian rhythm. The sleep-wake homeostasis or the circadian clock controls the sleep timing. It may have the greatest significance and greatest effect on the sleep of an individual. Sleep timing means the time you sleep and the time you wake up.

The circadian clock is also an inner time keeper, temperature controller, and an enzyme regulator. It is the rhythm that determines the ideal time for a person's restorative sleep and rest. It works together with a neurotransmitter called Adenosine.

Adenosine is a neurotransmitter responsible for inhibiting bodily processes involving wakefulness. Our circadian rhythm is commonly affected by poor sleeping habits such as overnight shifts, shifting time zones like flying from one country to another,

When a person goes to bed to rest, he or she undergoes a bodily and organized process called sleep. An individual passes through five phases of sleep: stages 1, 2, 3, 4, and REM (Rapid Eye Movement).

These stages progress into a cycle from stage 1 to REM. The cycle may be repeated more than twice in one night. An individual spends about 50% of his sleeping time in stage 2 of the cycle, 20% in REM and 30% is spent on the other part of the cycle. Infants on the other hand have different percentages wherein they spend about half of their sleeping time in REM.

Stage 1 is the stage in between sleep and wakefulness. A person's sleep would be easily disrupted if the person is in this stage. Muscle activity is still constant and the eye movements are still observed.

For the stage 2, the person's sleep gradually deepens. It is harder to wake a person in this stage of sleep.

On stages 3 and 4, a person no longer responds to environmental stimuli, Stimuli includes loud noises and bright lights. It is the stage where the person stays before progressing to REM.

REM or Rapid Eye movement is part of the sleeping stage which a person enters approximately 90 minutes after sleep is initiated. The deepest stage in the sleep cycle and is the hardest time to wake up a person.

Muscle activity is greatly reduced but the brain activity is noticeably highest. EEG tests confirm that a person's brain activity during the REM stage is similar to that when a person is awake.

Chapter 2:

Sleep Deeper, Wake Better

Synopsis

Still tossing around in bed even though you turned in a couple of hours ago? Do you feel uncomfortable and something keeps on bothering you every time you close your eyes? It may be that your circadian rhythm has been disrupted or certain factors have been affecting your sleep time.

There are different ways for a person to be able to sleep comfortably and wake up refreshed the next day. According to the National Sleep Foundation, you have a better chance of sleeping better and deeper when you follow the following:

Schedule, Exercise, Stimulant avoidance, relaxing before sleep, sleeping until sunlight, don't lie in bed, room temperature control, and consultation.

Sleeping Better

Setting a schedule means setting your sleeping time every night and waking up at the same time every morning. Setting the time helps your body adapt to the schedule and allows your circadian rhythm to work properly. Disruption in the sleeping schedule may cause sleeping problems or lead to insomnia. Keeping the schedule up during the weekend will also be beneficial to the person because they will not have any problems adjusting to the new routine on Monday.

Exercising has been seen to affect a person's sleeping schedule. Exercising for about 20 to 30 minutes a day often helps people sleep better at night. Exercise has been seen to help in releasing hormones needed for sleep. It is also beneficial for a person to exercise in the afternoon or 5 to 6 hours before sleeping. However, exercising right before sleeping will no longer be beneficial for the person involved.

Avoiding caffeine, nicotine, and alcohol to have a good night's sleep all have the same reasons. It affects the individual's sleeping pattern. Caffeine is a substance commonly found in coffee, chocolate, soft drinks, non-herbal teas, diet drugs and some pain relievers. Caffeine stimulates the brain and when the brain is stimulated, it would be hard for the individual to be able to sleep properly. Smokers tend to sleep lightly and often wake up early in the morning due to nicotine withdrawal. Alcohol robs the individual of deep sleep and REM sleep thus making the person wake up in the middle of the night.

Relaxing before bedtime allows the brain to slip into sleep quicker and allows deeper sleep. A warm bath, relaxing atmosphere, reading and even putting on music make it easier for the person to fall asleep. Creating a relaxation ritual paired with correct sleeping schedule will definitely allow a good night sleep. Also, sleeping until sunlight can help in the routine. Sunlight or bright lights helps the body's biological clock reset itself every morning.

When you are unable to sleep, lying in bed and doing nothing will not do you any good. Do something else by reading a book, listening to music, watching television until you feel tired helps. Lying in bed and not doing anything increases a person's anxiety thus reducing the chance for a person to be able to achieve deep sleep. Controlling room temperature provides comfort. If it is too warm or too cold, you would not be able to sleep properly or deeply. Experts suggest that having the right temperature will help you sleep nicely.

When still having trouble sleeping and the previous suggestions are not applicable, it is best to consult your doctor or an expert for that matter. Your physician would be able to help you. Remember, sleep is an important part of your day. To lose it means losing the day ahead.

Chapter 3:
Sleep That We Need

Synopsis

When you go to be tired bed and wake up refreshed the next morning, this only means that you were able to get enough sleep. But when you wake up with a heavy feeling, it only means that you either did not have enough or too much sleep.

A person needs to sleep. Sleeping is the main way of debriefing and resting and it is encouraged. Like all things that are needed, it must also be limited.

Physical activity that a person can perform sometimes is affected by how much time a person was able to sleep. According to studies, sleep can greatly affect a person's ability to function in a day. A person lacking sleep may not be alert enough to be able to function properly and may commit greater errors as compared to that of a person who had enough sleep the previous night.

What You Need

The optimal amount of a person's sleeping time can be determined by age as well as how well their circadian rhythm is functioning. Our optimal sleeping time is at its highest while we are young and slowly decreases when we age.

For a newborn baby, a child below one month old, they are in need OF12 to 18 hours of sleep on average. They need sleep greater than they need to be awake.

An infant, a child who is still under one year old, is in need of 14 to 15 hours of sleep. Toddlers on the other hand (aged 1-3 years old), are in need of 12 to 14 hours of sleep. Sleep at their age is needed for continuous growth and development.

Pre-schoolers (aged 3-5), are in need of lesser amount of sleep at 11 to 13 hours. When they reach the school age (aged 5-10), they are only in need of 10 to 11 hours of sleep.

For adolescents (aged 10 to 19), the optimal time for sleep is decreased to 8.5 to 9 hours.

Adults need about 7 to 9 hours of sleep per night. This amount of time is also applicable to the elderly. Having an exact amount of sleep every night means that your circadian rhythm is working perfectly.

Your circadian rhythm helps in keeping your brain and body functions in check. It is considered your very own body clock. It makes sure that you are awake on the time that you should be and asleep when you need to rest.

Aside from the correct amount of sleep that a person must get every night, experts also suggest that individuals must make time to take a nap in the middle of the day or right after lunch.

A nap after lunch is greatly advantageous because your brain function decreases after you eat a meal. It is due to the fact that most of your blood pools or is used by your digestive system thus reducing blood and oxygen supply to the brain.

According to studies, taking a nap during the day has been seen to decrease coronary mortality which is possible due to reduced stress to the heart when body functions are decreased when sleeping.

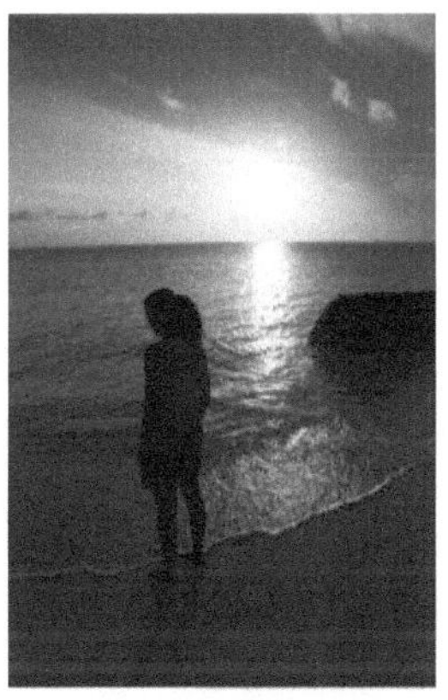

Chapter 4:

Insomniac's Deal

Synopsis

Been tossing and turning in your bed lately? Do you have trouble keeping your eyes shut at night or even falling asleep? Does a little sound outside your window jolt you awake? You might want to check it out because you might be suffering from insomnia.

Insomnia or sleeplessness is a sleeping disorder characterized by a person's inability to fall asleep or stay asleep as long as they want to.

Insomnia may be considered a sign or symptom and may accompany several sleep, medical and psychiatric disorders.

Insomnia can occur at any age. Insomnia can cause functional impairment to a person who has been experiencing these symptoms.

Insomnia

Insomnia is classified into three groups: transient, acute, and chronic. Transient insomnia has the shortest time. It usually lasts for less than a week and it can be caused by another disorder, changes in sleeping environment, timing of sleep, severe depression or by stress. An acute insomnia, on the other hand, is the inability to sleep consistently for less than a month. An individual is unable to maintain consistency despite adequate opportunity and circumstances for sleep. This may result in impaired daytime function. Acute insomnia is also called short term insomnia or stress related insomnia. Chronic insomnia is a type of insomnia that lasts for more than a month. It may be a primary disorder or caused by a medical or psychiatric disorder. Their effects vary according to its cases and severity. Effects may include fatigue and hallucinations.

Among the most common ways of relieving insomnia are Cognitive Behavior Therapy (CBT), Pharmacological and alternative treatment. Cognitive Behavior therapy is a therapy directed towards improved sleeping habits without using pharmacological help. In this therapy, patients are taught ways to improve sleeping habits and relieve counter-productive assumptions about sleep. It allows the person to take control of his sleeping and waking habits, giving them power and making them realize that it is up to them to help themselves.

Pharmacologic treatments include benzodiazepines, non-benzodiazepines, antidepressants, antihistamines such as diphenhydramine, and melatonin to improve sleep. Each medication prescribed is given according to what the person needs. Combinations of the drugs may be given if it is needed. The use of pharmacological treatments is oftentimes discouraged by physicians due to the possibility of tolerance and dependence of a person to a drug.

Tolerance means the body would need increased dosages of the drug because the initial dose is no longer effective. Dependence is when the individual would resort to medicine use even though it is not needed. Doctors and physicians nowadays create ways to limit the side effects of the drugs by decreasing the dosage when the person is able to sleep on his own.

Alternative treatments make use of herbal treatments in lieu of medications. The use of milk, teas, and other relaxation techniques has been suggested by experts. Milk has a sedative effect which can help an individual fall asleep better. Teas and herbs such as chamomile, valerian, lavender and hops have been introduced to the public and are seen as a better alternative than medications.

Chapter 5:

Energy Boosts from Short Exercises

Synopsis

It is a fast paced world that we move in nowadays. No matter how much we try, demands on our time would always become our problem. We no longer have time to have fun, relax or even have a long break that we deserve. These demands may take a toll on both our body and mind. We may later on feel physical or mental fatigue. Experts say that in order to stay fit and healthy in a demanding situation, we must create ways to ensure that we remain fit and mentally sturdy.

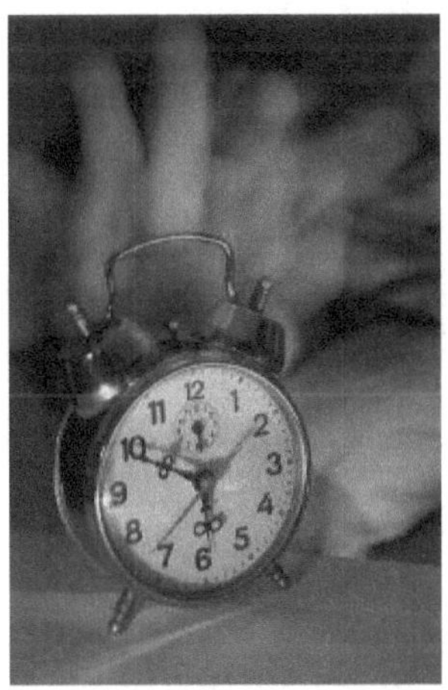

Energy

Exercise is a great way to fight stress, reduce fatigue, and increase our everyday energy levels. Even a few minutes spent on stretching those biceps and flexing those hamstrings can certainly help develop that. Studies have shown that there is a direct relationship between exercise and easy fatigability. Physically active people are more likely to have reduced risk for fatigue as compared to physically inactive ones. Exercise was also seen to have an effect towards the energy level of people with chronic illness like cancer and heart disease. An additional 15 minute walk in their routine is said to increase their capacity to deal with fatigue and stress.

The trick, as experts have said, is exercising when you feel tired. Tired people are less likely to put on their sneakers and go for a run or take the stairs instead of the elevator. Even a little increase in your activities can be helpful. Little exercises can be included in your routine without wasting much of your time. You can walk to work or ride a bicycle if it is a considerable distance instead of taking your car or taking a cab. You may also climb the stairs rather than take the elevator. Experts say that climbing the stairs for two minutes is equivalent to a 15 minute jog.

Also, making sure that you create a routine for you to follow will also help in the long run. You are able to know how many minutes you have left if you want to really go for an exercise of a different magnitude. Consistency must be maintained so as not to disrupt any major part of your routine.

For people wanting to perform short exercises, a simple run can be continued with a few minutes of stretching, curl ups and pushups.

The whole body must be stretched properly as to prevent any pain or irritation after the exercise. You may also do a couple of pushups and curl ups. You may also perform a couple of weight lifting activities but be careful not to over exert yourself too much. Also, for people wanting exercises that are easy to follow, a few minutes of instructional yoga, kick boxing, aerobics and other instructional exercises may be effective for you.

It is always good to remember to have some time to yourself. And it is always good to spend that free time on taking care of yourself and improving. A few minutes of exercise will always go a long way if you want to be as fit and healthy always.

Chapter 6:

Boost energy with Healthy Diet

Synopsis

Having a healthy diet is necessary to every human's everyday life. Whatever your reasons are for doing it, you are doing the best thing for yourself. It can be that you aim to lose weight or maybe you plainly want to have a life that is free from any kind of sickness and ailments. Having a daily healthy diet will definitely give you what your little heart's desire.

What most people have is a busy kind of lifestyle and in order to keep up with everything they need the right type of energy providing foods.

What other people may not be aware of is that your energy is boosted with a healthy diet. If your usual diet consists of processed foods or those that are greasy and straight from takeout counters, you are depriving yourself from the nutrients your body needs.

Good Diet

Having a healthy diet allows you to have a body in tip top shape and far from diseases which makes you weak. If you consume a balanced diet daily, you will live an active and energetic life. Not all people have the same dietary requirements and preference. Some may need to lose more weight and must be in a diet program which should be strictly followed.

For some, when diet is mentioned, what automatically registers in their mind are the unflavorful dishes they need to eat which causes them to quit dieting. Although there are dietary programs which may require less salt and sugar, there are also a lot of nutritious foods that can be consumed.

Fresh fruits and vegetables are always the first on the list. As the saying says, "An apple a day keeps the doctor away". Apples, oranges, bananas and other tasty fruits are always the best nutrient providing foods and energy builders too. You just have to continue eating them daily for you to have a fit body.

Healthy food allows your body to function perfectly including your blood flow. Avoiding unhealthy foods means no dangerous cholesterol inside your body as well as the excess fats which slow circulation. With everything that is working as it should, there is no reason for you to be weak and slow moving. You will be full of energy and all charged up because of what you have in you.

Variety is also a good way to keep your body fit. Learning about other foods that provide useful nutrients will allow you to enjoy living a healthy life. Eating the same kind of fruit everyday will lessen your interest with what you are doing. But if you come up with a variety of dishes that contains nutritious ingredients, you will even love the experience more.

Focusing on what you want will allow you to reach your destination. With a body full of energy, you will be able to fulfill everything that needs to be done. Who would want to live an unhealthy life that is full of worries and sickness? A healthy body is a healthy mind and when you have a healthy mind mistakes are lessen therefore success should be near.

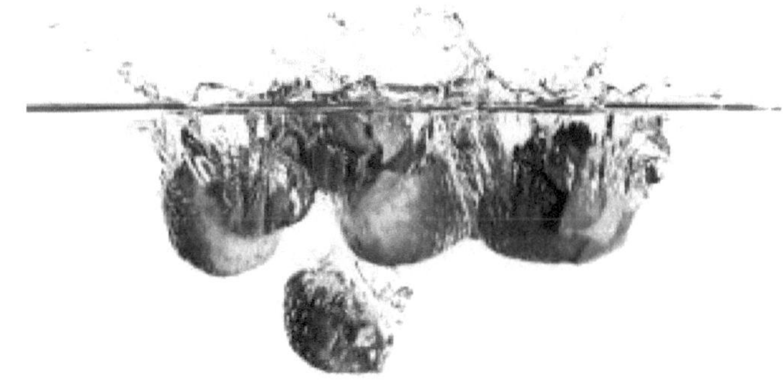

Chapter 7:

Set your mind's alarm clock

Synopsis

Normally, people rely on alarm clocks if they want to wake up early. It seems that it is impossible to be awake at an early hour without any use of any electronic or those technical devices and gadgets which have alarms. People are normally dependent on clocks not to be late for meetings, school and work but they should know that there is a better way to set an alarm on a particular hour without the use of any kind of watches or clocks.

The word "biological clock" may be something you have heard of before. This is the internal clock of human beings which tells the body to sleep when it is time to sleep or get up if it's time to wake up. The same with animals, they also have biological clocks which they follow every day making them wake up exactly the same time every day. The problem with our biological clock though is it has a lot of barriers making it "not work" the same way as how it works on animals.

Biological Clock

These are still our capabilities and abilities that hinders it to work properly overriding its ticking. But with serious focus and practice, we can use our own mind to set our mental clock. This may sound uncommon but it can be done. For sure you have met someone who wakes up the same time every day unless he is sick and needs to stay in bed to rest.

That is exactly what will come out of you if you program your mind to think that way. Just channel your mind into something you want done and it will naturally cooperate. Of course there are some preparations that need to be considered if you want to succeed and be able to have an operational mental alarm in you.

If you want to be able to do it, you may follow these steps.

1. First, you need to be in bed early free of noise and interruption. Your main intention here is to relax yourself and give it a good rest your mind to focus on your intention.

2. Set your mind and body in a relaxing mode. It would be easier if you start from one part to the other starting from the top. This method is also known as "entering the alpha level". You need to breathe deeply and start making your whole body relax. You will know if you are able to reach that state since your mind will

not be occupied with anything else. It takes practice though but doing this daily will make this process a lot easier as well as faster.

3. Think of somewhere you would like to be when you want to relax. That will allow you to keep yourself calm and relax.

4. Picture a clock set in a particular time you want to wake up. It can be any kind of clock or watch as long as it is the one that you fancy.

5. Command yourself to wake up at that particular hour you set your mental clock to and you will wake up the next day on that very hour.

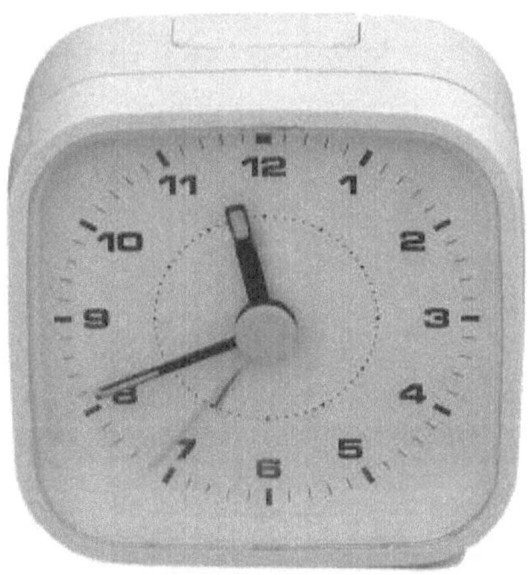

Chapter 8:

Practice meditation before sleep and after wake up

Synopsis

Sometimes with all the issues in life and things to keep up life becomes similar to a roller coaster ride. Having all these in your mind, you tend to stay in bed all night fully awake and having a hard time putting yourself to sleep. You should never deprive yourself of sleep and a good rest, without having that, you will wake up the next day feeling down, cranky or impatient. This is not something healthy for you, your family and your work.

With so many things on your mind it is impossible for you to relax even during the time you close your eyes. There are people who fix on little things and consider them a life threatening situation if it is undone which causes them to stop relaxing even if there is a need to do so. These are people who even worry about things if their backs are already touching the bed.

Meditation

You need to understand how important sleep is and you must submit yourself on practices that may reward you with a chance to prioritize daily rest and good night's sleep. If your mind always floats back to your issues at work or your family problem even if your body is already telling you to sleep, maybe it is time for you to start meditating.

Pressure is what keeps your mind wandering off instead of getting to rest. Practicing meditation can truly provide you with the solution your body needs. Taking sleeping pills is not a healthy option since it can be dangerous to you if you become addicted to them. Meditation on the other hand will allow you to have a good sleep.

Practicing meditation before sleep and also after waking up will allow you to have a relaxed mind. It may be a little difficult when you are still starting but as you get used to it, it will work like magic.

It always starts by preparing yourself for your intention. Giving yourself a relaxing bath and making your whole body calm by massaging your arms, hands and all the other parts of your body which you feel stressed and tired.

When you finally feel your entire body is comfortable and nothing feels stiff you can sit down on a chair with your back straight. Let your feet touch the floor firmly and then close your eyes taking long and steady breath in and out of the nose. Repeating this three to five times will help clear what is in your mind.

When you are freeing your mind from all your worries you can breathe in slowly counting to three and then breath it out counting up to six and do this breathing pattern seven more times.

After this, lie on the bed with your stomach touching it with your arms folded and cheeks resting on them. Just focus on the rising and falling of your breathing and allow your mind to dwell on that relaxing moment.

Once you have gotten used to this, you can also try just sitting down while you meditate and relax yourself. Doing this daily before sleep and when you wake up will absolutely free your mind from stressful concern. A healthier happy you will come out from it too.

Chapter 9:

Managing stress the smarter way

Synopsis

Have you ever seen a successful corporate executive who does not look slick and stress free? Rarely can you tell when they are stressed out and that is because they expertly learned how to successfully manage the level of stress they are in. They are smart enough to know that if they walk around in a disarrayed state and let their subordinates see them that way, these people will also be affected or doubt their leadership capabilities too.

You do not need to be a corporate executive to be able to battle stress and appear great in front of people. You can actually find a way to eliminate your worries and stress producing concerns and live a happy life each and every day. You must first understand that there are two types of stress and be able to identify which is which. Eustress also known as positive stress is the type of stress we need for our health. The one we need to stop doing is called episodic acute stress.

Being Smarter

Stress in general is the reaction of the body by releasing a sudden energy burst which causes hormones to shuffle and this can be draining if it becomes too much. Eustress is giving you a positive effect since it makes you relax and allows you to feel positive such as bungee jumping, going out on your first date with a long time crush or just simply having a quick speedy slide down the ski slope. Anything that can make you feels the rush and makes your adrenaline pump.

Episodic acute stress on the other hand is the type that drains your energy with no positivity in it. Dwelling on an unfortunate event of your life or worrying about unpaid bills is one of them. If you are smart enough how to turn all these negatively causing issues into something that will become beneficial to you, you will be free from the stress that eats you up causing you to become unproductive.

Once you realize how to determine the type of stress you are in, you can easily find ways to remove or at least minimize the effects it will do for you. But in order for you to do that, you need to have a healthy mind to come up with working ideas. Living a healthy life is the key to this. Eating the right kind of food and doing exercise will allow you to live in this state of health.

Remember that the reason why you are in a stressful situation is because you were not able to foresee the events that caused it. If your

mind is clear from worries and useless concerns, you will have a backup plan to solve it in case it arises. The smart way to deal with stress is absolutely having a relaxed healthy life. There will be times that you will be affected by it because that is normal, but being resilient is something that you can be. A healthy mind will give you ideas to bounce back and get back on the race again.

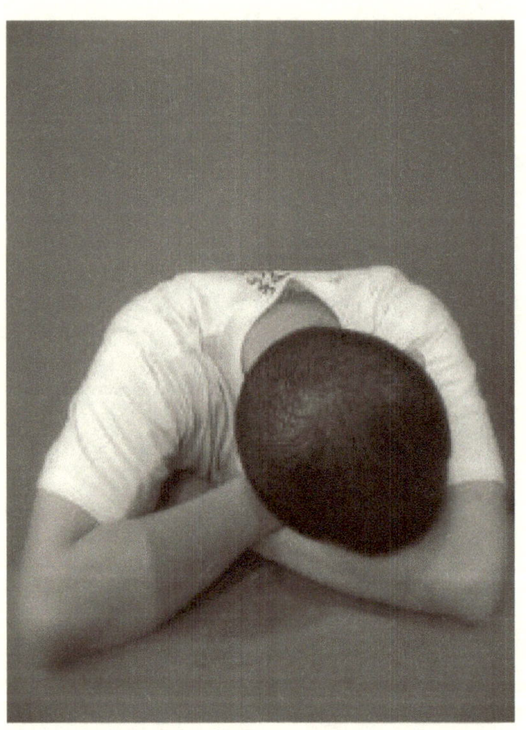

Wrapping Up
Making Manifestation a Permanent Habit

Not many people may have realized it but being enthusiastic in life gives you the power to change your life, positively. You can see things differently and give you the chance to accept and appreciate life even more. In return life will become a lot easier to live. Enthusiasm is the positive energy that drives you to reach your goal. Some people are driven by money, some by material things and by love.

These are the factors that motivate you and give you happiness in life as well as giving a whole new meaning to your existence. It is always present to everybody but only a few are able to use it for their good. Seeing everything in a positive way or allowing your mind to think that something good will turn out even after a huge blow will eventually lead you to your lifelong dream.

The most common factor that drives people to move forward is love and affection. It can be for your family, your parents, a girlfriend, a friend or for a pet. Doing everything for your loved one will give you a fire inside you that burns and let you "chug" your way up. It is a very powerful feeling that will allow you to think that everything will turn out right despite the hindrances and your limitation.

Enthusiastic people are positive people and are totally different from the rest. In the event that stressful issues and problem arises, most

people would show negative signs and turn cranky, moody and grumpy. But with the enthusiastic ones, they always find a reason to smile and be happy with a tiny possibility that might eliminate the problem at hand.

If you can make yourself that person, then you are on the right track. Your most anticipated success will be nearer and you will find that life is indeed great. Planning each day enthusiastically will allow you to appreciate everything that is in front of you. You would know what you will be doing the next day and thinking ahead will provide you with ideas that can turn it into a great day.

Having an enthusiastic life is living a healthy life. You won't have to think more about problems and other concerns that will put your spirits down since your mind will permanently have a reason to cheer you up. Inspiration works and it can be anything that can motivate you. Inserting motivating activities in between your responsibilities will allow your happy thoughts keep on flowing.

Simple things like calling home and checking on your family will give you happiness. If your heart's pleasure is drinking coffee after work then look forward to it. It doesn't have to be a huge thing before you consider it special. You simply have to make it your reason for smiling and everything will fall into place. The next day will be all happy and gay if you plan it to be one. Happiness can do wonders and you can be one if you live life enthusiastically.